T0090149

Wellness in the Parables through Meditative Poems and Prose

Trevor Moorley

Order this book online at www.trafford.com
or email orders@trafford.com

Most Trafford titles are also available at major online book retailers.

Printed in the United States of America.

ISBN: 978-1-4269-4197-9 (sc)
ISBN: 978-1-4269-4198-6 (hc)
ISBN: 978-1-4269-4199-3 (e)

Library of Congress Control Number: 2010912864

*Our mission is to efficiently provide the world's finest, most comprehensive book publishing
service, enabling every author to experience success. To find out how to publish your book,
your way, and have it available worldwide, visit us online at www.trafford.com*

Trafford rev. 09/20/2010

Trafford
PUBLISHING®   www.trafford.com

North America & international
toll-free: 1 888 232 4444 (USA & Canada)
phone: 250 383 6864 ✦ fax: 812 355 4082

Contents

FOREWORD

God made man and woman in His image as His special creation. But the image of God in mankind was marred when Adam and Eve sinned in Eden. Since that time, the human family, made as an indivisible unity of body, mind, and spirit continues to share this fallen nature and all its consequences. Because of sin, achieving the fullness of wellness and well-being have been seriously undermined.

Jesus Christ came to redeem fallen humanity and restore the image of God in us. He used parable teachings extensively as an effective method in reaching humanity with the gospel. All the parables have rich truth that are not evident on the surface, but are revealed only as one digs below the surface.

Wellness in the Parables through Meditative Poems and Prose goes beneath the surface and provides for us the amazing truths found in the parables. It is written to help us grow in understanding the challenges of our existence here on earth. Trevor Moorley has done an amazing job of compiling the parables in meditative poems and prose, presenting them in a way that is concise, practical, and useful.

This book is not only a valuable resource item for both clergy and layman, but also for all of the human family as it presents a blueprint of principles of which to live by as we face the everyday struggles of life.

Lucious Hall,
Senior Pastor and Pastoral Counselor; Former Speaker,
Voice of Hope Radio Broadcast, Florida, USA.

PREFACE

I have discovered that deep within the parables of Christ are experiences that are designed to make us whole. Men and women are crying out to be made well again in this world of depravity and selfishness. These parables provide a wellspring of wellness principles and may just be the answers to many of our wellness concerns. Every parable in its own way reflects some measure of wellness toward experiencing abundant life here, and in the hereafter. The way we relate to God, to our selves, and to others impacts significantly on personal wellness. I like how Travis, J. W., & Ryan, R. S. (2004) in their *Wellness Workbook* consider *wellness* as the "integration of body, mind, and spirit–the appreciation that everything you do, and think, and feel, and believe has an impact on your state of health and the health of the world."

Authorities on wellness consider it an active process through which we can become aware of and engage in choices that will accentuate a more successful existence. Such a model will incorporate six basic dimensions–social, occupational, spiritual, physical, intellectual, and emotional. For maximum benefit, each area should be integrated with the others, and thus, we need to consider wellness in each area to be holistically well.

A careful study of the parables will impact our attitudes positively and shift our focus from hopelessness to meaningful living. I have reconstituted these parables into meditative poems and encouraging prose. Remember that they are earthly stories with heavenly meanings and we should be careful not to misinterpret their messages. For example, the parable of the Ten Virgins was not intended to mean that in the Church fifty percent of the members are wise and fifty percent are foolish. Or, in the parable of the Rich Man and Lazarus, that all rich men will go to hell while all poor men will go to heaven.

I encourage you to read in a spirit of mindful meditation and internalize them so as to achieve your wellness fulfillment.

This book can be helpful in your personal devotion, in-group discussions, in skit/drama/recitation presentations, or even as a treasured gift to a friend. May your hearts be blessed as you receive this word with gladness.

ACKNOWLEDGMENT

To God, the Father, God, the Son, and God, the Holy Spirit for their guidance in knowledge, wisdom and understanding.

To my devoted and supportive wife, Radica, for her constant encouragement.

To my son, Trevis, and daughter, Tremaine, for their love and inspiration.

To you, my dear reader, for your desire to seek knowledge that will make you truly whole.

Candle Under a Bushel
(Matthew 5:14-16; Mark 4:22, 23; Luke 8:16, 17)

You're the light of the world, if you will
To show others light along the way,
Just like a city that's perched on a hill,
Its brilliant glories there to display.

No man sets a candle brightly alight
Then hides it under a bushel so—
But raising it well to sufficient height,
'Tis light for all with house aglow.

Let your light so shine before other men
That your good works they'll surely see,
And glorify your Father who is in heaven,
That they too may shine for eternity.

Light and darkness simply cannot co-exist. The presence of one implies the absence of the other.

It is amazing that God considers us as little lights to shine in such a way that others may develop a love for Him and for His eternal kingdom. In other words, we have a royal calling from the King of kings and Lord of lords to be active partners in His majestic dynasty. And not only do we have a royal calling, but also a dynamic enabling since He supplies the power to provide the light as long as we remain "plugged in" to Him.

There may be those who would desire to extinguish your candle and create adversity by striking at your self-worth, self-concept, and self-esteem. But grab your match of values, connect to the Source of light, the Creator God, who said, "Let there be light" in the beginning, and there was light. And so, light up again! Let none steal your joy.

The apostle Peter reassures us that "ye are a chosen generation, a royal priesthood, a holy nation, a peculiar people; that ye should show forth the praises of Him who hath called you out of darkness into His marvelous light." *(1 Peter 2:9, KJV).*

Why not share your light today with a pleasant smile to someone, or an encouraging word, a listening ear, a small deed of kindness even. It may just brighten their day with thanks to God for you. You will experience the joyous satisfaction of emotional wellness springing up in your heart as you reach out to others to help brighten their day.

Wise Man/Foolish Man
(Matthew 7:24-27)

Like a wise man who builds on solid rock,
Is to hear God's Word and obey willingly,
While the rains descend with a mighty shock,
And the fierce winds beat so mercilessly.

His house stands firm, so safe and sound
In spite of wind and storm and rain.
For its foundation is built on solid ground,
And anchored deep in solid terrain.

But he who fails to hear and do,
Is building on shifting and sandy soil.
For the floods will come and the hurricanes too,
And this house will crash in great turmoil.

It makes good sense to pay particular attention to the structural integrity of your foundation as you engage construction of your building. Earthquakes, hurricanes and other forms of natural disasters may wreak havoc causing buildings with their poorest foundations to collapse or suffer more extensive damages than others with appropriate and adequate preparation.

Even heavy traffic using roads with poor foundations causes such roads to quickly deteriorate and can therefore become a nightmare for road users.

Like the physical, so the spiritual. A strong spiritual foundation is essential for developing resilient characters toward withstanding social pressures and emerging victors in our spiritual battles. Spiritual wellness crowns our efforts as self-responsibility and love take their rightful places.

As such, some tried and tested foundational ingredients include daily prayer, study of God's Word, and sharing your faith. Indeed, the apostle Paul reminds us that "we wrestle not against flesh and blood, but against principalities, against spiritual wickedness in high places. Wherefore take unto you the whole armor of God, that ye may be able to withstand in the evil day, and having done all, to stand." *(Ephesians 6:12,13. KJV).*

Unshrunk Cloth on Old Garment
(Matthew 9:16; Mark 2:21; Luke 5:36)

Threadbare and torn
Old and outworn
The garment's almost gone.

To patch the tear?
With new cloth there?
Will not improve the wear!

The old is the old,
The new is so bold
Cannot be hot and yet be cold.

Simple modification,
Without character transformation,
Will surely breed destitution.

Wellness is borne of a free choice. It is the privilege that each of us possess and has the right to exercise as we seek optimal health. It is neither an endpoint nor a static state, but a dynamic process incorporating varying degrees or levels of wellness. Ryan & Travis (2004).

New Wine in Old Wineskin
(Matthew 9:17; Mark 2:22; Luke 5: 37, 38)

Think again, and again.
New wine in old bottles is in vain!
A loud explosion 'twill generate:
Broken pieces will accumulate.

But think again, this is true,
New wine is saved in bottles new.
For the new wine's index of expansion
Therein allows for its preservation.

Many times we have to make radical changes in our lives so as to move forward onto our goals. Now, heaven should be our ultimate goal and we should understand that we are just pilgrims on this earthly journey. So, we should place more emphasis on wholesome lifestyles today - physically and spiritually – in preparation for a new tomorrow.

Our self righteousness is like filthy rags. There is nothing inherently good within us to recommend us to Christ. But surrendering to Christ allows Him to transform us and give us new meaning to living. The apostle Paul notes in 2 Corinthians 5:17, KJV "therefore, if any man be in Christ, he is a new creature: old things are passed away; behold, all things are become new." So the sinful evil practices that engaged our lifestyle and may have brought hurt to ourselves and to others, will now cease in favor of righteous deeds by the grace of God.

It is not merely applying "spiritual cosmetics" just to look good before God and others, but a radical mind and heart transformation initiated and maintained by the indwelling Holy Spirit of God.

Newness in Christ is a blessing of wellness in demonstrative love to God and to fellow human beings.

The Sower

(Matthew 13:3; Mark 4:3-9: Luke 8:5-8)

Into the fields for a day of toil,
The farmer scattered seeds upon the soil.
Hoping in his heart for a bumper crop,
He kept on sowing and would not stop.

But oh! some seeds on the wayside fell,
The hard and beaten path, you sure can tell,
And with haste the birds these seeds they ate,
Giving them no chance to germinate.

Upon rocks and stones with little earth
Some seeds were blessed with little growth,
But with a scorching sun and no depth of root
They withered and died before bearing fruit.

Among some thorns some seeds got there,
They grew a while and were about to bear,
But entangling thorns as a yoke-like cloak,
Obstructed growth and the plants did choke.

Yet towering high were plants so tall
From seeds which on fertile soil did fall,
With a blooming, bountiful harvest at maturity
To nourish and bless all of humanity.

This world is made up of people with varying mindsets. Some have absolutely no relish for things spiritual or for the Creator God. Such are simply satisfied to eat, drink, make merry and die. They may reason that after death, whatever happens, happens...

Then there are some with good intentions for heaven and home at last and gladly receive God's Word. But for whatever reasons, personal situations or external circumstances, they become unmotivated, losing their focus and their faith. Social pressures seem to overwhelm and consume their wellbeing so that spiritual victories are elusive to them. The past, with its brokenness and guilt, seems to act like a fetter to the feet preventing forward movement. There is an enslavement of sorts, like those entangling thorns in the parable. The life seems crushed and the satisfaction of wellness threatened.

But there is hope. Jesus can fertilize your seemingly barren soil and see to it that you produce bountifully. His voice echoes with love in Matthew 11:28 KJV "Come unto me all ye that labor and are heavy laden, and I will give you rest."

Then the prophet Hosea encourages us to "sow to yourselves in righteousness, reap in mercy; break up your fallow ground: for it is time to seek the Lord, till He come and rain righteousness upon you."*(Hosea 10:12)*

An Enemy Did This
(Matthew 13:24 - 30)

The kingdom of heaven is likened to a man
Who sowed good seeds with the very best plan,
But while he slept, quite unawares
Among his wheat an enemy planted tares.

As the grains appeared on the stalks of wheat,
The tares just hindered, they being counterfeit.
'Sir, didn't you sow good seeds?' his servants cried,
'From whence came these tares all side by side?
We cannot allow these tares to stay,
We'll uproot them now and throw them away!'

"Oh, no," he replied, "you may not get it right,
You may destroy good wheat, compounding the plight.
Just let them grow until the harvest time
When the wheat shall be in its fullest prime.
Each then will be separated without mistake,
The tares will be fuel for the fire's sake.

Sowing faithfully for God is bound to provoke the wrath of Satan, the enemy. He will work subtly and stealthily to thwart the best of plans. He has a way of mixing truth with error so skillfully that for a while one may not be able to distinguish one from the other. But as the saying goes, 'the longest rope has an end.'

When someone sabotages my good work, how is my wellness response in such areas of feeling angry, being angry, feeling sad, or conflict resolution and so on? How do I maintain my dignity?

With the passing of time, truth will emerge as error is exposed. It takes patience to wait on the Lord, commitment to surrender to Him and faith to let Him fight some of the battles that we are unable to undertake.

At the appointed time, according to God's reckoning, all wrongs will be vindicated and all injustice will meet with His justice. Sometimes by taking matters into our own hands, we may act in such a way that a bad situation becomes worse. This is not to say that every obstacle, challenge or problem is to be shelved in waiting for the good Lord to do something about it.

With our God-given intelligence, in partnership with His will, interpersonal conflicts should be resolved in a spirit of reconciliation as far as humanly possible. At other times we may have to abide and wait on the Lord, trusting Isaiah's counsel that "they that wait on the Lord shall renew their strength.... they shall run and not be weary; and they shall walk, and not faint." (*Isaiah 40:31*).

The Mustard Seed
(Matthew 13:31, 32)

Consider God's kingdom a mustard seed,
The tiniest of the tiny, of a seed indeed.
But when a man sows it in his precious field,
The abundance of profit is an amazing yield.

From a tiny seed to a powerful tree,
The landscape is awesome, oh, what majesty!
The birds of the air find refuge and food,
A rest for the weary, reviving the mood.

It is amazing how some things considered puny and insignificant maybe, can be transformed into formidable products. This excellence may occur under favorable conditions of nurture. But even under trying physical and social conditions with all the hostilities and aberrations in life, the grace of God can help you develop your 'insignificant' talent for His glory and honor.

The mustard tree spreads and blooms for the benefit of the environment. It is not selfish in this regard. We too, need to bloom for the Lord so that others will be blessed.

This parable sends us a powerful message that we need not think of ourselves so small that we cannot achieve great heights under God. He is able to make the seemingly impossible possible. We are talking of the One who parted the Red Sea such that a whole nation could walk through to the other side. Our thought patterns impact our sense of wellness and our sense of wellness influences our thinking. There is this circular relationship which needs to be explored well.

It takes surrender *to* Him and focus *on* Him. Jesus himself said, "... with men it is impossible, but not with God: for with God all things are possible." *(Mark 10:27, KJV).*

Goodly Pearls
(Matthew 13: 45)

A jeweler by trade,
Specializing in pearls, good pearls,
Authentic, top of the line!
Been travelling far and wide,
Keen eyes and a sense of feel.
Profit yes, but customer satisfaction too.

Ah, wait! This one is rare!
Exquisite!..... a priceless gem!
Incomparable! A chip of the heavenly foundation?
Unbelievable, absolutely precious.

He must have it, indeed, indeed,
At whatever honest cost.
So he sells all his personal valuables,
All his possessions; sacrifice beyond compare....!
Just so he can purchase it.
It won't be traded... Never.... no, never!

The sacrifices we sometimes make to acquire earthly goods may be understandable given the deep sentimental values we attach to such goods. We are sensitive to things of value; we recognize irresistible bargains and we go after them with unrestrained zeal. Do we, really? Maybe.

In many cases, selfish immediate gratification is a mere driving force. In others, it is simply to keep up with the Joneses. But in some cases, there is sincerity in the sacrifices to acquire the goods because of appropriate personal meanings attached to them. In terms of your wellness outlook, do you contemplate what is meaningful to you and regularly reexamine your values and priorities? Have you considered the difference between what simply pacifies and what really satisfies? There is much room for discussion here at this point, I must admit.

Today, likewise, many have discovered that personal joy and satisfaction of embracing Jesus as their personal Savior from sin. They are making tremendous sacrifices along their faithful journey in preparation for His soon coming kingdom.

Some have given up jobs, income, friends, fame and fortune in order to hold on to the precious reality of eternal life in Christ. This assurance can be yours in response to the blessed invitation recorded by John, "And the Spirit and the bride say, Come. And let him that heareth say, Come. And let him that is athirst, come. And whosoever will, let him take of the water of life freely." *(Revelation 22:17, KJV)*.

The Treasure Hid
(Matthew 13: 44)

Wait a minute!
I just can't believe it. ...
Digging for yams, lo and behold! ...
Is this really my pot of gold?

It must have been here for ages now,
Undiscovered, protected, sheltered somehow.
My Lord, my God, what indescribable joy!
Enough praises my tongue fails to employ.
This field looks abandoned, apparently,
Yet it harbors such riches efficiently....
You know what! I'll hide again this priceless treasure
I shall buy this field for my life long pleasure –

"Realtor, sir, what is your price?"
"Only a thousand, friend, and the price is nice!"
"Realtor, sir, this field is surely my deepest need,
Please let me have it, with you I earnestly plead,
I have sold all my possessions, both great and small,
Got me nine ninety-five and here is all."

"My friend, where there's a will there's always a way,
Consider the field yours, you can have it today."

Many temporal possessions today simply exist to pacify our lives – fancy cars, houses, education, money etc. But Jesus in the life, not only pacifies, but truly satisfies!

Searching the Word of God is like digging up that abandoned field. Many today are neglecting to spend quality time with the Word because of so many distractions and preoccupations. They do not find the treasure because the searching is absent.

This treasure represents Jesus Christ and His love to us. His love is more precious than gold. He is the answer to all our perplexities. He is our refuge in the time of storm, the wind beneath our wings to bear us up, the King of kings and Lord of Lords.

Nothing should be considered too valuable to surrender in order to get hold of His love. All He asks for is our sin-polluted hearts in exchange for His rights to rule in our hearts that we may experience the peace of God that no amount of money or temporal possessions could ever purchase.

This is Wellness, my friend.

Jesus himself said, "Search the scriptures: for in them ye think ye have eternal life; and they are they which testify of me."*(John 5:39)*

Net Cast in the Sea
(Matthew 13: 47)

The kingdom of heaven, just spare this thought,
Is like a net that's cast into the sea.
All kinds of fish in it are caught ...
Some big, some small, some trying to flee.

The fisherman labors quite patiently
By night and by day in the ocean's deep,
Exposed to the weather, yet faithfully
For a rewarding catch he hopes to reap.

When the net is full he comes to shore,
The good fish he chooses for him to use,
Casting away the bad and what's impure
The good ones, keep; the bad, refuse.

So shall it be at the end of the world,
The angels will perform a separating job,
The righteous will gather in God's holy fold,
The wicked destroyed with Satan's mob.

Not everyone who is shouting and singing for Jesus and talking about heaven is going there. The sad truth is that many are aboard this gospel fishing boat, but not all will make it as chosen of God to reach the heavenly port. The word of God says that "many are called, but few are chosen."*(Matt.22:14)*.

Simply put, practicing contrary to what you are preaching obstructs the harmony between wellness and communication. The messages we reinforce through our self-talks should focus on increasing our genuine wellbeing.

There is going to be a separation – one group for eternal life and the other for eternal damnation. There will be no middle ground. The responsibility is ours today to "make our calling and election sure" and not to neglect so great salvation.

1 John 1:9 assures us that "if we confess our sins, He (Christ) is able to forgive us our sins and to cleanse us from all unrighteousness."

The Ten Virgins
(Matthew 25: 1 - 13)

Again the kingdom of heaven, I want you to know,
Is likened to ten virgins dressed so spotlessly white,
Waiting for the Bridegroom, enthusiasm aglow,
Lamps in their hands for light in the night.

But five were wise in thought and in deed,
And five were foolish, too complacent maybe.
The wise had extra oil in case of need,
The foolish failed to prepare for any emergency.

The Bridegroom did tarry for long was the wait,
And slumbering and sleeping were the virgins all.
The minutes ticked on as the hour got late,
When at midnight they heard a resounding call.

"Behold the Bridegroom cometh, he's getting very close,
Get ready to meet him and welcome him in."
With haste off the floor they all quickly arose
Trimming their lamps for more light there within.

'Twas a very, very sad and unfortunate plight
For such a grand occasion of pomp and pride:
The lamps of the foolish refused to light
Their vessels were dry; no more oil there inside.

"Give us of your oil," to the wise they said,
"Our lamps are out and we cannot miss the event."
"Not so," they replied, all shaking the head,
"Ours may run out too, with the same predicament."

"Why don't you go to the store and buy?
Someone around may be willing to sell,
You should've had for yourselves abundant supply
Just as we did as you surely can tell."

They searched the streets for some oil, in vain,
All shops were closed in the dead of night.
Their hearts in sorrow and their feet in pain,
Darkness all around for that lack of light.

While they were searching with hope getting dim,
The Bridegroom arrived with his jubilant lot.
Those who were ready went in with him,
And the door was shut... securely shut.

Shortly after were frantic knocks on the door
Pleading and crying, voices broken somewhat,
"Lord, let us in, we are sorry evermore"
Sadly he refused them with "I know you not."

Again, two classes of people are presented here. The five wise virgins represent one class of people who are well-prepared, fortified, diligent and serious about their calling and responsibility. The oil, which represents the Holy Spirit of God saturates their living. They carry extra oil in case of emergency. In other words, the have an extra infilling of the Holy Spirit's power attained by submission to Christ and demonstrated in joyous service to others – a measure of wellness in the life.

The fruit of the Spirit, love, is manifested in unmistakable degree. So too are the attributes of love – joy, peace, patience, goodness, temperance, faith *(Galatians 5:22)*. True Spirit-led folk will not settle for mediocrity in service but will constantly seek to improve on their God-given talents for His glory and the benefit of others. This is one way of stocking up on extra oil in the life that can be accomplished. When the ultimate motive is to glorify God and not self, the 'peace that passeth all understanding' is anointing to the soul as God multiplies your blessings.

The five foolish represents that class of people who are failing to make adequate spiritual preparations and will eventually rob themselves of their heavenly home when Jesus, the Bridegroom, returns. They will be lost not for the unavailability of oil, the Holy Spirit, but because they were too complacent, thinking that today's grace is sufficient for tomorrow's. They are contented with 'raindrops' of grace when they should be pleading for 'showers' of blessings.

They are happy to provide 'one mile' of service to others when they have the potential to provide 'two miles.'

The Bridegroom's delay that tried their characters revealed that they were wanting or they fell short in true character development even though they appeared externally impressive as well-dressed virgins.

Today, the King of kings, Jesus, is apparently in delay of His promised soon return for His prepared and faithful ones. We need to use this time wisely to be spiritually fortified and energized while waiting for Him. More prayer, more power. More Bible studies, more knowledge. More surrender to Him, more love for Him. More love for Him, more service to others.

And the principles of true wellness in the life will begin to unfold.

John 14:1 -3, in Jesus' own words say "Let not your hearts be troubled .... I will come again and receive you unto myself, that where I am there ye may be also." The apparent delay is just to help us get ready. Do not miss out on it, for it may be too late for some when the door of mercy is shut. When Jesus returns, that prepared group will be welcomed in while the unprepared will be left out much to their anguish and destruction. Accept Christ today, tomorrow may be too late.

The Unforgiving Servant
(Matthew 18:23–35)

He came to the king with tears in his eyes,
A pathetic poor figure with not much of a size.
"Ten thousand you owe me and you must pay right away,
But somehow I feel that you simply will not pay.
So your wife, your children, and you will be sold,
To repay me my money, its worth in pure gold."

"I'm sorry, my lord, things are really, really rough,
So many bills to pay, and life is truly, truly tough,
Have patience, good lord," he begged on his feet,
"I promise, dear lord, my commitment I'll meet."

"Somehow I'm moved with compassion for you,
I want to release you to start your life anew.
So here I forgive you of this burdensome debt,
Go in peace, dear friend, no longer to fret."

Smiling with joy, he left well-relieved,
Forgiven by the king, just can't be believed!
As he walked on along, his brains a bit dense,
He met a fellow servant who owed him a hundred pence,
He grabbed him by the throat and shook him violently,
"Pay me what you owe me.. now!..... immediately!"

With tears in his eyes on his feet he did fall,
Begging for patience with a promise to repay all,
But the man refused and cast him into prison,
Until the debt be repaid whenever the season.

His other fellow servants were all moved to tears,
So they went to the king and expressed all their fears.
The king was annoyed when he heard what was done,
He commanded that unjust man in before the set of sun.

"A big, huge debt I forgave you therefrom,
Yet you cast one in prison for a much smaller sum,
I had compassion on you in your desperate time of need,
Couldn't you do likewise to a lesser indeed?"

"So now in prison I'll surely have you cast,
There's a lesson to learn for you there at last.
Forgiveness was sweet when I gave it to you-
Really, you are forgiven as unto others you do."

Nothing was wrong with that servant requesting his hundred pence from his fellow servant. The issue was that having himself being forgiven of more than a hundred times that little debt owed by his fellow servant, he would proceed to cast that little man into prison without returning the kindness.

Given the circumstances presented, that servant went unjustifiably overboard–to the extreme. He did not share with his friend the patience and love freely expressed to him moments before. In so doing he failed to experience a healing deep in his soul, a healing that would have championed socio-emotional *wellness* and *well being*.

Was it a 'temporary superiority complex' issue, having regard to the fact that he had just emerged from the king's presence? Or, was it because of a heightened adrenaline rush with money now consuming his mind? Whatever it might have been, he forfeited a golden opportunity to pass on the grace and kindness to a poor and helpless fellow being.

How many times we get brutally harsh against a brother or sister who offends our delicate sensibilities with somewhat trivial issues. Yet we rejoice when we have made some serious blunders against others and they graciously forgive and reassure us that "we are all in the same boat," or, "we're all climbing up the rough side of the mountain together."

Exacting our due pound of flesh with arrogance and so-called righteous indignation may very well lead to our spiritual downfall and physical ill-health. We may need to learn how make the intelligent choice from among the good way, the better way, and, the best way of doing a good thing. Think about it.

Let us pause and consider two issues;

1. *In what ways can I design a lifestyle so that I may achieve the highest potential for my wellbeing?*
2. *How can I practice loving acceptance of myself as a demonstration of the wellness process?*

The Ten Talents
(Matthew 25: 14–30)

Like a man on a journey
Into a far, far country
Is the kingdom of heaven.
He calls in his servants one by one
To leave them something while he's gone.

"Chief servant, here's five talents for you,"
"My next loyal friend, here I give you two"
"My next trusted friend, I leave you one."
"While I am gone out there at large,
Do your best; you're all in charge."

Away on business he attends,
Contacting several of his friends.
And a long time passes by ...
Then he heads for home with a passionate zeal,
For familiar experiences his to feel.

Reckoning time for his servants three,
As he calls them in so dutifully
So that they can talk.
"Tell me boys, what did you do
Since I bade you guys fond adieu?"

"Here's the five you gave, with five more gain.
I did not waste my time in vain
Neglecting opportunities so grand."
"Well done, well done. Enter into my joy!
I'm so proud of you, my special boy."

"Your two yielded two," the other chimed,
"That's four in all and it's so well-timed
For your welcome home."
"Well done, well done. Enter thou into my joy!
I'm so proud of you, my special boy."

The third showed up with the one he got,
Not an extra dime, since invested not,
For negligent was he.
According to their abilities was each his share
To plan and to use with skill and care.

"I was scared of you, Lord, I want you to know,
Thinking you reaped much where you did not sow.
And I buried your talent…"
"Rascal, the bank would have kept it safe and sound
With interest too!… instead of the ground."

"Cast him out, bind his hands and feet,
To weeping and wailing, and gnashing of teeth,
And utter darkness."
He that produces much, much more will he get,
But slothfulness and neglect will cause your regret.

While the talents here in this parable have economic implications – whether gold or silver to be traded for profitable returns – the lesson is clear that the businessman Master expected dutiful diligence from his entrusted servants.

He recognized the capabilities and abilities of them all. They were not all the same, so he gave unto them according to their abilities. His focus was not so much on quantity of return as on quality of input.

Complacency, slothfulness and neglected opportunities are character destroyers and wellness robbers that retard or destroy spiritual growth.

God has given to each of us talents or skills, money maybe, or even provided opportunities for us to grow in His grace and be of service to others in a bid to advance His coming kingdom. Some are more endowed than others, but we all have something we can invest for the Lord so that His name can be glorified. And in the process we ourselves may find fulfillment in our daily lives.

For one, each of us has the talent of time in the same measure – twenty four hours in the day. How do we spend it? Invest it? Everything belongs to God; we are mere managers of His goods and will be called upon to account for our managing one day. Even our bodies belong to Him. Some say "this is *my* mouth, I can say what I want." The truth is you can do it – but the day of reckoning may find you gnashing your teeth in that same mouth. No one wants that bitter experience.

Wellness is a balanced channeling of energy – energy received from the environment, transformed within you, and returned to affect the world around you.

Laborers in the Vineyard
(Matthew 20: 1– 16)

Now the kingdom is like a householder,
Who at 6am sharp sought laborers to hire.
Into his vineyard to plow and to sow,
That a bountiful harvest surely will grow.
When they agreed for a penny a day,
He sent to the vineyard to work right away.

Around nine or so he went out again.
At the marketplace stood some idle young men.
"Go to my vineyard and work today,
Your price will be fair at the end of the day."
With joy they accepted as all did agree
To work for the Master as best as could be.

At the marketplace again at noon and at three,
He found more men standing so idle and free.
"I'll pay you what's right if you work today,
You'd be well-satisfied with your take-home pay."
Dashing off to work with a glint in their eyes,
They hastened to work for that pleasant surprise!

Then at five in the evening for another visit there,
More idle men were standing right in the square.
"Why sand ye idle here all the day?" he cried,
"Because no man hired us," they all replied.
"Go to my vineyard, I'll pay you what's right,
It's one hour's work before the start of night."

When the night did come at the set of sun,
"Twas six o'clock and the long day was done.
He called in the workers to have them all paid,
For they all did their work and they all obeyed.
The last hour's workers got a penny for the day,
Much more than expected, didn't know what to say!

The ninth to the three each got a penny too,
And wild with excitement not knowing what to do.
The first came along hoping to get more indeed,
But each was given a penny as they all had agreed.
They murmured about the one-hour workers' pay
Equaling theirs who bore the burden of the day.

So he reasoned with them in a tender, loving voice,
"My friends, I did no wrong, for it was your very own choice
To agree with me for a penny a day.
Please accept your due and gently go your way;
I am fair and good, and lawful and just.
Remove greed from your lives, be such one can trust."

God is fair and just. He keeps His promises to us with a faithfulness that is generally not akin to us human beings.

Some people respond faithfully to the call of God to be servants of His high and holy kingdom in the teenage years. Others respond in early adulthood, and even others in late advancing years of life.

But the gratifying consolation is that at whatever stage or station in life one accepts the Lord and is faithfully obedient to Him and His commands, he or she is assured of the same promise of eternal life with Him. Enduring to the end is what counts.

The workers in the parable started off at various times of the day but they all endured until nightfall or the end of the day. They stuck to duty, making the best of their opportunities. This brought self determination and inspired an embracing of usefulness – qualities of wellness in the workplace.

At the end of the day, my dear friend, you may be able to identify with the apostle Paul when he said,

"I have fought a good fight, I have finished my course, I have kept the faith: Henceforth there is laid up for me a crown of righteousness, which the Lord, the righteous judge, shall give me at that day: and not to me only, but unto all them also that love His appearing." *(2 Timothy 4: 6 – 8).*

Your Wellness hope that'll make you cope...

Sorrow looks back,
Worry looks around,
Fear looks down,
But Faith looks up.

The Two Sons
(Matthew 21: 28 – 32)

What do you think ...
About a man with two sons?
Says he to one ...
"Go work in my vineyard today."
And his response?
"No, I will not."
But his conscience bothers...
He repents, and quickly goes to work.

Says the man to his second son:
"Go work in my vineyard today."
"Oh, sure I will," he assures.
And then what?
He does not go. ...
And he really does not go.
Just a matter of words,
Or, is it?

For one, disobedience in word
But, obedience in act.
For the other, obedience in word
And disobedience in act.
Who will the father favor?
Who has integrity?
Actions do speak louder
Than words.

This earthly life provides many lessons for our learning in preparation for our heavenly life. Our thoughts, words, and actions do not always synchronize. Sometimes to say 'No' is quite appropriate and so too is it in saying 'Yes.' But to say 'yes' when the intention is 'no' and vice versa implies deceit and mistrust.

While temporary benefits to the ego might accrue, worthy character development may be short-changed. The child of God is guided by a conscience surrendered to the Holy Spirit and the practice of righteousness integrity is always the focus. The Spirit's enabling power strengthens the feeble and willing heart.

It is reassuring to know that the The Holy Spirit of God comes to our aid to guide us. Isaiah 30:21 tells us *"And thine ears shall hear a word behind thee, saying, This is the way, walk ye in it, when ye turn to the right hand, and when ye turn to the left." KJV.*

The Wedding Feast
(Matthew 22: 2 – 14)

Hosting a special feast for his only son,
Special friends were invited to share in the fun.
The king's servants pleaded with them to appear,
But none would come to demonstrate their care.

Those special guests the king planned to treat
With lavish preparations no other could beat
Hoping that they would surely change their mind
And come with joy, so gracious and kind.

Other servants pleaded from door to door,
'Preparations in place, so much food galore,
Come in to the marriage and do not delay,
You're specially invited, do not stay away.'

With laughter and scorn they refused outright,
Choosing business and pleasure and fun in the night.
Some held the servants and hurt them physically,
Others went so far as to kill them mercilessly.

On hearing the news the king became annoyed,
He sent his army and the murderers were destroyed,
Their city was burnt to ashes on the ground,
No ungrateful aggressor was there to be found.

Then new invitations were extended to the poor,
Those destitute, marginalized, and hungry to the core,
Their wedding garments provided all free of charge
As they came so thankful in numbers so large!

But when the king came in to his great astonishment,
He saw a guest seated without his wedding garment,
"Why are you not wearing my precious wedding robe?"
But speechless was he to his Majesty's probe.

"Bind him hand and foot and take him far away,"
He commanded his servants, in such utter dismay.
"Into outer darkness, again I do repeat,"
There shall be weeping and wailing, and gnashing of teeth.

For many are called but few will be chosen,
Is this special lesson of the kingdom of heaven.
Invitations from the King demand your acceptance,
For eternity at last shall be your inheritance.

Generally, people would consider it an honor to be the guest of royalty. Some would give anything and make tremendous sacrifices to be in the presence of a celebrity or head of state and so on. To intermingle with dignitaries is a coveted feature of many a personal agenda today. They eat, drink and sleep it with a consuming passion.

In this parable we wonder why did the rich folk refuse the king's invitation, even going so far as to beat and kill some of his servants. What are the lessons to be learned?

Firstly, the king represents Jesus Christ and He is the King of the universe; we are all his servants.

Secondly, He invites us to come to Him so that we can experience the fullness of joy in Him and be saved by His grace. The symbolism of marriage is the sense of belonging to Him, accepting Him as Lord of our lives.

Thirdly, the wedding garment is His robe of righteousness that covers our nakedness and unworthiness. We cannot make ourselves righteous since all our righteousness is like filthy rags.

To start with, Jesus on earth had no celebrity or secular dignity status. His birth was too lowly. He had no pedigree backing. To accept an invitation from Him was below the dignity of many rulers of His day, and even today. In Mark, chapter 10 and verse 23, Mark notes that "how hardly shall they that have riches enter the kingdom of God." And again he observes that it is easier for a camel to go through the eye of a needle than for a rich man to enter the kingdom of God.

Yes, there are many rich men who are faithful to God and will be saved. But in the main, the deceitfulness of riches is a stumbling block preventing many from making a full surrender to Christ.

Secular business, worldly pleasures, and personal perceptions of salvation by self-righteousness take precedence over responding to Jesus. Even religious prejudice and radical extremism can become so inflamed that violence is considered justified by some in settling religious differences. Accepting the wedding robe is symbolic of accepting the righteousness of Christ for a covering of our unrighteousness and social prejudices. It is free of charge, just for the asking and receiving. This is life-changing, life-giving, life in abundance, with healing and holistic wellness incorporated.

The less privileged in society tend to be more responsive to the invitation of King Jesus. That man who wore his own garment instead of the king's, even though he accepted the invitation, represented a class of people who say yes to Jesus but is desirous of salvation on their own terms and not on Jesus'. Some of their own terms may be good works, transcendental dynamics, or reengineered theology with no biblical basis.

The Bible plainly states in *Ephesians 2:8 "By grace are ye saved through faith and that not of yourselves; it is the gift of God."* Nothing of ourselves we do can merit our salvation. Only Jesus saves. It is His gift to us. We simply accept. In the Book of Isaiah 1:18 we read *"Come now, and let us reason together, saith the Lord: though your sins be as scarlet, they shall be as white as snow; though they be red like crimson, they shall be as wool."*

Why not confess your sins to Jesus right now in private, accept Him as your Savior from sin and walk away rejoicing in His love?

The Fig Tree
(Matthew 24: 32 – 44)

Now learn a parable of the fig tree
Examine its growth with care.
Things you know by what you see
Should teach us much in life so dear.

When the branch is soft and very slender,
Place your finger there round about.
The branch is oh so really tender
As tiny leaves are growing out.

This is a sign that summer is near,
As always happens without a fail.
To see, to touch, to smell, to hear
Signs of conditions that prevail.

Signs of the times do surely endorse
The Christ of an impending summer.
His soon return is even at the doors,
'Tis something we must remember.

No one knows the day as such,
Not even the angels high above.
But signs of the times do tell us much,
That we should show more Godly love.

Some signs before that widespread Flood
Were revelry, gluttony and infidelity,
Serving the flesh, little time for God,
It's no different today, in reality.

Only eight were saved in that blessed ark
Together with some animals of choice.
The majority died in the waters so dark
Refusing to heed the Preacher's voice.

Two groups at the time of the end,
One will be saved; the other lost.
One will live with Jesus their Friend,
The other destroyed; didn't count the cost.

As structural changes in the fig tree of Bible times pointed to an approaching summer, so changes in the social conditions of the world were to be signs pointing to the second coming of Christ.

The Bible refers to some changes that will take place so as to give us an idea of this great momentous occasion when He shall come to receive His faithful followers. Matthew chapter 24 cites the frequency of natural disasters-hurricanes, tornadoes, floods, earthquakes and so on, the intensity of international political conflicts, physical environmental changes, and social upheavals on planet earth.

The apostle Paul writing to Timothy also supports these predictive signs while focusing on man's inhumanity to man. This world is reeling under the scourge of diseases like AIDS and cancer, for example. Human injustice and sinfulness are increasing in alarming proportions. So often the wrong is deemed to be right, and vice-versa, much to the dismay of law-abiding citizens.

Something stupendous is about to happen. It is the blessed appearing of our Lord and Savior Jesus Christ in power and great glory. We need to be ready for the event now since there will be no second chance then.

The ability to discern the signs of the times today with their prophetic relevance greatly contributes to personal wellness as individuals seek to actively chart a way forward to inspire meaning to their daily living.

Spread the Wellness all around that it may very well abound....

Words of kindness are as welcome as the smile of angels...

The Wicked Husbandmen/Laborers
(Mark 12: 1-12)

Acres of vineyard a certain man planted,
Hedged it around as you would've expected.
Machinery in place for manufacturing too,
Buildings erected-what a fantastic view!

To some laborers he rented his vast acreage,
Before setting out on a grand pilgrimage.
He then sent a servant for rent that was due,
But they beat and chased him, empty-handed too.

Again another servant went to them instead,
They stoned him till there were wounds to the head,
He had to flee, so battered and bruised,
The rent for their Master they ungratefully refused.

Yet another was sent for his rent to get,
But they made sure he met a horrible death.
Some others they beat so mercilessly,
And others they killed so disgracefully.

Deciding to send his only begotten son,
Thinking they'd respect him, each and everyone.
But with torture they violently killed him there,
Hoping for the inheritance if they killed the heir.

What then shall the Master come and do?
He will surely destroy those laborers too!
And give out the vineyard to honest laborers,
Faithful and true in all their endeavors.

One great lesson in this parable is that God is the owner of everything and that He has placed us here on earth to manage His goods faithfully. The rent that was called for symbolized a call to obedience to God through His servants, the prophets and messengers.

Jesus was teaching that many would slight God's call to such an extent that they would presume to physically hurt them. Indeed history testifies of the persecution and martyrdom of many Bible-believing followers-Jerome, Huss, Wycliffe and Martin Luther, just to mention a few.

The only son in the parable was a direct reference to Jesus Himself who would not only be persecuted but tortured and killed as well. Again history bears record of this.

The last part of the parable ends in victory in that the vineyard will be kept by worthy laborers as the unworthy will be destroyed. In other words, God's kingdom will be populated with obedient, faithful and worthy believers – people who have love and respect for self, others and God. Understanding this through this parable should intensify our personal *wellness* that will be evidenced in our human to human interactions. We will be more tolerant and loving instead of spiteful, prejudiced and abusive.

The Absent Householder
(Mark 13: 33-37)

For the Son of Man is verily
A man undertaking a far journey
Leaving his home, indefinitely.
To his servants he delegates authority,
Everyone, some responsibility.

A special request to the gatekeeper:
Be on the lookout for the Master,
For he may return sooner than later,
Evening, midnight, daybreak, whenever.
Stay awake; it may be that very hour.

Be ready, you never know when
Your Lord will come again.
Keep the faith, all women and men,
Watch and pray to your Lord and Friend,
And a helping hand to others lend.

As pilgrims on this earth, we are travelling daily amidst troubling and perilous times. The distress and pains that constantly undermine our potential wellness need to be banished forever.

The promise of Jesus in John chapter 14 verses 1-3 is certain: *Let not your heart be troubled... I will come again.... I go to prepare a place for you; and if I go to prepare a place for you, I will come again and receive you unto myself that where I am there you may be also.* As with the parable of the fig tree we need to be alert and responsive to the signs of the times that signal His soon return. Matthew chapter 24 enlightens us very well with these signs.

We need to be on guard for His return lest He returns and finds us unprepared. Yes, we may stumble and fall down at times on this rugged journey, but He encourages us to get up again, shake off the dust, seek His forgiveness and keep moving forward.

His grace is sufficient for us. He is always a prayer step away from us on this journey. Talk to Him about your troubles, trials, joy and victories- talk to Him as to a friend. He cares for us and loves us so much such that He does not want any of us to perish but that we will come to repentance and accept His offer of eternal life. Be ready!

The Growing Seed
(Mark 4: 26–29)

Like the kingdom of God, is some seeds in the sod,
That a man did cast, in the winter's blast.
Then he goes to sleep, while the seedlings peep
Out of the earth, and much to his mirth.
Yet he does not know how these seedlings grow.

The earth feeds the roots, then an abundance of fruits!
But first comes the blade, then the ears are made,
And the corn is full, so very plentiful.
So with sickle in hand, combing through the land,
The harvest is due.... with celebration too.

Wellness that's tried and in your heart will abide...

Love the Lord with all your heart,
To others more love impart,
Plants and animals crave your love also,
And loving yourself, see your wellness grow!

The Creditor and Two Debtors
(Luke 7: 41-43)

"Simon, Simon, I want you to hear this."
"Speak Jesus, not a word I'd wish to miss,
I promise you my undivided attention
To inspire my heartfelt meditation.'

"Two debtors to their creditor were summoned,
The first owed 500 pence, and 50, the second.
But both had absolutely no money to repay,
They were sad, forlorn and in total dismay.

Then the creditor graciously forgave each debt,
Hence, no more pain, anxiety or fret.
With relief they walked out the door.
So who do you think will love him more?"

Simon paused and pondered in his heart,
"I suppose he who was forgiven the greater part."
"Rightly so, Simon, and in every instance,
Forgiveness brings joyful deliverance."

The greater the debt forgiven should invoke the deeper appreciation. However since forgiveness cannot always be quantified thusly, this statement cannot be a hard and fast rule or law. The principle involved here though is that when one cancels a heavy debt, whether financial, relational or both, the gratitude factor from benefactor to the one gracious enough to release that burden should be unmistaken.

The truth is Jesus has released us from the burden of eternal death by canceling that debt when He paid with His own life on the cross of Calvary almost two thousand years ago. The Bible records that *"The wages of sin is death, but the gift of God is eternal life through Jesus Christ our Lord." (Romans 6: 23)*.

Because of sin, we were destined to die – not the sleep in the grave when we are buried or cremated – but the eternal death by virtue of hell's consuming fire. However, the release from this death (and debt) is available just for the accepting of Jesus as our personal Savior from sin.

Accepting Jesus into your life by surrendering to His call demonstrates our great appreciation for His loving sacrifice on our behalf. Revelation 3: 20 says of Jesus, *"Behold, I stand at the door and knock. If any man hears my voice and opens the door, I will come in to him and sup with him."* He will not force us. The choice is ours.

The Good Samaritan
(Luke 10: 30—37)

"And who is my neighbor? And from what social class?"
Queried the young lawyer, with such a face of brass.
Then Jesus taught him this parable
Of a man in some really big trouble.

A certain man left Jerusalem for that great Jericho
For whatever the reason, we may never know.
But step by step, his was a relaxing walk,
All by himself and with no one to talk.

Then out of the blue some bandits appeared,
Who stripped him and beat him and left him for dead
At the side of the road all penniless and in pain,
And bleeding and groaning from blows like rain.

By chance a certain priest came driving his expensive ride,
He simply glanced at him and passed on the other side,
While saying some prayers in his righteous, holy mind,
That God will send someone who is helpful and kind.

Then another church elder came by that very place.
He stopped and looked at his sore wretched face,
But with a mortal fear of compromising his pride,
He, too, passed by on the other side.

But a Samaritan "dog" on his humble little ass
Was journeying too on that road to pass.
But on seeing that victim in such horrible mess,
His heart was touched with deep distress.

He went up to him, his wounds to dress,
Pouring oil and wine as he cleaned up the mess.
Then on his own humble beast he strapped him straight
And brought him to an inn so as to recuperate.

He stayed up all night as a friend indeed,
For a hapless poor stranger in desperate need.
Himself in need and desperately poor,
But with a willing heart to do something more.

The following day he must depart hence,
So he gave to the host a grand two pence,
Saying, "Take care of him, and should you spend anymore,
When I return, I will repay you for sure."

Which of these three are you likely to agree
Is a neighbor to that man in his wretched misery?
"He who showed mercy," the lawyer guessed
"Well, go and do likewise and you will surely be blessed."

The experience of meaningful social wellness will not allow the "good Samaritan" in each of us to be selectively bias or operate from a point of "total convenience only." One might be tempted to assume that had the victim been a priest or church elder, or someone in a high station in life maybe, the issues of bias and inconvenience displayed by those men of the clergy may have disappeared in favor of positive intervention to assist the brother.

Again, it may not have been convenient to reschedule commitments, change directions, or accommodate the needy in your expensive car. "Good Samaritan" responsiveness on the way to the heavenly kingdom will demand of Christ's followers the eradication of social class discrimination when welfare duties call. Service should not be solely limited within the walls of the church but extended to the wider community as love in action.

A good motivating counsel is found in Matthew chapter 25 and verse 45. Jesus himself is speaking, "....*Inasmuch as you have done it unto one of the least of these, you have done it unto me.*"

A Wellness point that will not disappoint…

Exercise is beneficial in treating some back-aches, ulcers, arthritis, insomnia, nervous tension, indigestion, asthma, diabetes, anxiety, and low-level depression. It truly is a wonder 'drug'.

A Friend in Need
(Luke 11: 5—13)

Your cupboard is bare
Not a morsel to spare,
Things are really, really tight,
And your good friend visits at midnight.
Weary, weary feet,
And needing something to eat,
A place to sleep,
And a secret to keep.

So to another friend you go over
At that very midnight hour.
"Friend, I know it's late,
But I cannot wait.
My friend is visiting now,
He must eat, somehow.
Lend me three loaves, I beg of thee
To feed my friend, this is my plea."

Shall he refuse?
And make some excuse?
The door is already shut...
Trouble me not...
Children in bed...
Sleep's in my head...
My wife is ill,
She just took a pill.

No, no, not at all.
Because of his friend's unusual call,
And the state of affairs,
His concerns and cares...
He rises with glee
To cancel his misery,
By supplying the bread
So that friend can be fed.

So, ask and you will receive,
Seek and believe,
Knock and wait,
'Twill open by faith.
If your son asks for bread,
Will you give a stone instead?
Or, if he asks for fish,
Give a serpent for his wish?

Or, if an egg is his cry,
Will you a scorpion supply?
You will not think of it,
No, not one bit!
So uncharitable though we be
We treat our children graciously,
How much more shall our Heavenly Father give
The Holy Spirit to us who shall ask and believe.

The destitute friend is confident that he can approach his neighborly friend at any time with the assurance that he has enough to supply and *will* supply. This blessed friend is sympathetic and ready to respond as the need arises. The social support network here is so strong that social wellness is amplified in both their lives. One finds fulfillment in life willing to lend a helping hand; the other, grateful for the benevolence of a dependable friend.

So it is with our Heavenly Father. We should have the confidence to come boldly to the throne of grace through prayer knowing that our God can "supply all our needs according to His riches in glory." *(Philippians 4: 13).* The communication channel of prayer to God is open 24/7.

Eat a variety of grains daily, especially whole grains. Keep white rice, pasta, starches, and sweets to a minimum. Drink sufficient water daily and get some mild sunlight. Do not over work and engage some regular deep-breathing exercises in the open air. Get sufficient restful sleep, have a connection with God and a positive attitude to living.

The Rich Fool
(Luke 12: 16—21)

The rich man's ground produced so bountifully,
He stood amazed at the abundant yield.
As far as his eyes could possibly see,
Were millions of grains on his expansive field.

To himself he says while beaming with pride,
I'll demolish these barns and bigger ones build.
My fruits and grains in them I'll hide,
What a windfall I have from the soil I've tilled!

I will say to my soul: relax with ease,
You shall stash away goods for many, many years.
Eat, drink and be merry and do as you please
For rich now you are, so banish all fears.

But God had a word for that covetous soul,
He was to die that very, very night:
He will not live to become very old,
Selfish in motive and trusting in might.

Rich in the world yet poor in God?
Laying treasures on earth and none above?
Better poor today and be covered by the blood,
Sheltered by His grace, protected by His love.

We do not know what the very near future holds for us. The fortune tellers, psychics, parapsychologists and the like, may reveal some things but they do not make them authorities on knowledge of the future. Or else they will be winning every lottery ticket in town! Only God knows the future, your future included. Within the next twenty four hours you can possibly lose a friend, your home, or your life. Who knows? But God.

We may be richly endowed now, today—but we can lose it all in a flash—to some unexpected environmental disaster.

So why not reduce your stress level by living one day at a time. Why spend excessive anxious hours seeking to selfishly expand and jealously protect material increase when socioeconomic vulnerabilities loom desperately large today? While you may cite Biblical quotes that money is a defense and it "answers" all things, you must remember that it is also transient and temporal. That is, it only will last for a period of time. On the contrary, your soul's salvation is of eternal consequence. As such, we need to pay close attention to Christ's words, *"What shall it profit a man if he gains the whole world and loses his own soul?"(Mark 8: 36).*

The Faithful Servant and the Evil Servant
(Luke 12: 35–40)

Be dressed, be ready with lamps all alight,
Like men awaiting the Bridegroom at night.
As he comes from the wedding with that special knock,
They hasten to receive him as the door they unlock.

Blessed are those servants whom the lord shall find
Waiting and watching with alertness of mind,
For he may come in an hour that none can foretell,
And he'll reward their faithfulness so abundantly well.

If a landlord knew when a thief is due,
His name, and the time, and every other clue,
He would watch and be ready with a definite plan
To protect his house and get that rascal man.

Since you know not the hour of the Savior's return,
Be ready and watchful with a zeal to learn.
For in such an hour as you may think to doubt,
He may well appear with a triumphant shout!

Time flies….and someone dies,
Was once alive but had lost the drive,
Oppressed, suppressed,….distressed, depressed,
Opportunities came, didn't appreciate the game…
Wellness refused…illness, the accused.

The Faithful and Wise Steward
(Luke 12: 42–48)

Who then is that faithful and wise steward,
Whom his lord makes ruler over his household,
Who is so efficient regardless of the reward,
True to duty, to not be bought or sold?

Blessed is that servant, I hereby decree,
Whom the lord shall find at his arrival
Managing prudently with accountability,
Goods and services, all at his disposal.

He shall surely recommend his promotion,
For satisfied his soul shall be.
What faithful stewardship and devotion
Exemplified in diligent responsibility!

But the servant who says in his mind
My lord will not make haste to return,
Then he abuses his staff and gets so unkind,
Idle and drunk, his calling to spurn.

The lord of that servant may come at a time
When he is least expecting such.
He will fire him from his position sublime,
Ostracized, rejected, and kept out of touch.

The skills and talents that we all possess,
Are granted to us in degrees,
They're all to be used to uplift and bless,
To invest according to our abilities.

Who has more has a greater responsibility
Than the one who certainly has less,
For failing your test can cost your eternity
So be faithfully true in doing your best.

The Barren Fig Tree
(Luke 13: 6–9)

A certain man had a fig tree
That was planted in his yard.
One day he examined it carefully,
Expecting some fruits to be had.

So sad, the tree bore him none,
Three years of barrenness,
In spite of rain and air and sun–
It was a symbol there of emptiness.

Just occupying much needed space...
He told the gardener to cut it down.
But the gardener begged for one year's grace,
To dig and fertilize all around.

Should it bear, it will remain,
Otherwise, it will have to go.
So like us, if our life's in vain,
We just may lose it in one fell blow.

In the last three parables, discipline and productivity are themes that figure prominently and may very well embrace, to a large extent, the concept of financial wellness. The blessings that God provides in terms of the sun, rain, personal health and wealth and so on are to be used constructively for the welfare of man and our planet. It gives impetus to that adage that "living is giving and giving is living, and all things would die if only receiving." Someone told me a long time ago that the Dead Sea is so called because while it receives much from the environment, it gives back nothing in return. As children of God we need to produce some good fruits of love, patience, kindness, care and concern for others.

The Great Supper
(Luke 14: 16–24)

One of the greatest suppers in the land
Was organized by a certain man so grand.
He extended to many folk a special invitation
To come and dine in fine celebration.

The day for the supper his servant went
To fetch the guests for the grand event.
But they all with one voice sought to be excused,
Claiming reasons that you'd surely be amused.

The first said "I've bought a piece of land, you know
I must view it today, I have to go.
I pray thee, understand why I must refuse,
To look at my land is my legitimate excuse."

The second chimed "I've bought five yoke of oxen, you know
To try them today, I need to go.
I pray thee, understand why I must refuse,
To test my oxen is my legitimate excuse."

"Well, I've married a wife," the third exclaimed,
To view her? To try her? To be excused? None he proclaimed,
But with a voice of steel that made the servant numb,
He firmly declared, "I cannot come."

So the servant reported the disappointing news
Of the expected guests and why they did refuse.
The master was angry at their rejection,
For supper was ready with no one for celebration.

He dispatched his servant in an angry voice
"We need folk here to come and rejoice—
Go quickly out in the streets and lanes,
Bring the poor, blind and crippled in all their pains."

From the highways and hedges they all came along,
And the house was filled with a mighty throng!
The former invitees failed to count the cost,
Were successful in the world, but their souls were lost.

Matthew chapter 6 and verse 33 reminds us to seek the kingdom of God and His righteousness first and all these things (material necessities like food, clothes, shelter etc.) shall be added to us. God's formula for true success in life is He first, then me, followed by His blessings. Oftentimes we want to be first, God in second or third place, if at all, and still craving the blessings. The truth is, He still sends the rain and the sunshine on the just as well as the unjust. But accessing the fullness of His blessings demands that we place Him first in all our undertakings. We should talk to God in prayer before every major decision or commitment. Our plans for the day should be committed to Him first thing in the morning as we seek His guidance. Obedience to Him should be our highest priority.

The thing is, when the call of God comes laying claim on our lives, we offer so many excuses to avoid surrendering to Him. We are either too young, too feeble, not married, do not have a good job, or, the church is too boring and hypocritical and so on. The problem is that while we linger trying to sort out these concerns in our own strength we may die in our disobedience. And after death comes the judgment. What then? Why not surrender to Christ today and let Him sort out your concerns? Tomorrow may vey well be too late.

Relax those eyes by William Bates, MD.

1. *Sit or lie down and take a few moments to breathe deeply.*
2. *Now gently close your eyes.*
3. *Place the palms of your hands over your eyes, with your fingers crossing over your forehead.*
4. *Use memory and imagination to realize a perfect field of black. See it so black that you cannot recall anything blacker. Do not try to produce any experience.*
5. *Allow 2 to 3 minutes, breathing easily.*
6. *Remove your hands, slowly opening your eyes.*
7. *Do this several times a day, or whenever you need to relax.*

Building a Tower and a King Making War
(Luke 14: 28–35)

Why start a huge construction
Without first counting the cost?
Is there sufficient for completion
So that your efforts won't be lost?

Suppose after doing foundation
The finance is all gone,
Men will despise your calculation
And even laugh you to scorn.

Or which king to war will go
Not considering his resources well?
Whether peace may also calm the foe
And even serious conflicts quell?

If you wish my disciple to be,
You also need to count the cost.
Set your sight on eternity,
And in Jesus you must trust.

Living haphazardly with little or no aim and goals in life may result in you being tossed around, confused and unstable. And this can spell disaster for wellness in all its forms as directional focus becomes blurred or altogether lost. There is a high cost attached to low living; penny wise and pound foolish, maybe. This cost may be your emotional, financial, social, spiritual wellness or a combination of them all.

But really, have you counted the cost if your soul should be lost? You can talk to Jesus today without any further delay. It just does not make sense to trade eternity with Jesus for temporary mundane and painful pursuits.

The Good Shepherd
(Luke 15: 3–7)

One, two, three, ... ninety-nine.
I am missing one of mine!
It is now the end of day,
But one of my sheep is gone astray.
I need to find it immediately,
My God, just where can it be?

The shepherd searches so far and wide,
By rocks and rivers and rising tide,
Through thistles and thorns and precipice,
In the alleys and valleys, nothing to miss,
Calling its name with tenderness,
In the dark, chilling night of gloominess.

Out in the wilderness so far from the fold,
There's a weak, faint cry of the sheep in the cold,
He rushes to its aid though tired and weak,
'Twas hours of patience his own to seek.
He puts it on his shoulders with thankfulness
And carefully walks home with gentleness.

He calls to his neighbors with a triumphant voice,
Come along with me and let us rejoice,
For through the briars and thorns and rugged ground
My sheep that was lost has just been found.
Likewise joy bells ring in heaven o'er one repentant soul,
More than ninety-nine just persons who are already whole.

Jesus, the Good Shepherd, will do all in His power to save us, the sheep who keep going astray. Indeed, He gave His all, His very life, a ransom for us that we may be redeemed from the claim of eternal death because of sin.

The sheep, in its innocent adventure, lost its way by straying too far. Nightfall had crept up. Out there in the darkness and coldness bruised, battered and shivering was the sheep. It was vulnerable to the predators out there. It knew it was lost but could not help itself to get back home.

Sometimes we can see ourselves in that sheep, isn't that so? But Jesus comes in search of us down there in our desperate and helpless situation. He keeps calling like God, the Father did in the Garden of Eden, "Adam, where are you?"

We may think that we are too far gone but we must remember that while God hates the sin, He loves the sinner and is constantly reaching out to rescue and save. Do not resist, but gladly accept His offer of salvation today. Jesus and His angels will rejoice that you did!

The Lost Coin
(Luke 15: 8–10)

Yes, all her life's savings—
Ten pieces of silver!
What if she loses one piece?
Yes, one precious piece!
Insignificant?...To some, yes.
To others?...who cares?
To her?...still precious.
Cannot sleep, cannot rest,
It must be found!

She lights her candle,
Searches everywhere,
In the house,
Around the house.
She sweeps and checks
With a microscopic eye.
Lost, but still precious!
She must find it,
The search goes on.

Aha, in a far corner,
Amidst the dust
The coin is found!
The search was not in vain,
Rejoicing after pain!
She calls her neighborly friends
To rejoice too.....
So do angels rejoice,
When the lost is found!

The metal coin, by its nature, had no mind to know it was lost. To its owner it was lost, yet she had faith, patience and courage to search diligently until she retrieved it. Though lost, it was still precious and valuable to her.

Some people are so steeped in sin, consciences seared to such an extent that they fail to recognize their lost condition. But such are still precious and valuable to Jesus. And it may warrant His personal, divine, miraculous intervention to get their attention because He wants to retrieve and receive them unto Himself. He has a thousand ways to do this, but He may choose to have His faithful, patient and courageous disciples of today to seek out such for His everlasting kingdom. Time is running out and the search cannot be forever.

The Prodigal Son
(Luke 15: 11–24)

A certain man had two teenage boys,
In many ways he shared their joys,
But the younger got tired of staying at home,
A yearning in his heart to get out and roam.

To his father he went with a demanding voice,
"I'm leaving this house and this is my choice,
Give me my inheritance, to you I stress,
Cannot wait for your death; I'm young and restless."

Father beseeched him to change his mind,
But to good counsel he was deaf and blind,
So his father gave him his share of the wealth,
Which should've been due after his death.

A few days later and so anxious for the "game,"
The youth departed to seek his fortune and fame.
Into a far country, so far from home he went,
Wasting his life in reckless entertainment.

There came a time he had no money in hand,
And there arose a famine in that mighty land,
He began to be in want, became so destitute,
His friends forsook him—a rejected, homeless youth.

He sought for a job from nine 'till nine
But the only thing he found was to feed dirty swine.
Oftentimes he would wrestle the pigs for their feed,
For no man gave unto him in his hour of need.

From riches to rags how low did he fall,
With tears in his eyes back home he'd recall,
That his father's house had food and more to spare,
Yet he perished with hunger and his clothes threadbare.

So he rehearsed a confession his dad to tell–
"I have sinned before heaven and before you as well,
I'm no longer worthy to be called your dear son,
Please hire me as a servant, I'm so unworthy and undone."

Rising to walk with no shoes on his feet,
Penniless and wretched with a smell that wasn't sweet,
He started for home, full of shame and disgrace,
How in the world could he look on his father's face?

Even though he was gone for many a years,
His father remained in grief with pain and tears.
By night and by day he would look with eyesight dim,
Praying for a miracle of a son returning to him.

At a time when he thought all hope was gone,
A halting, limping vagrant contrasted the setting sun.
The distance was great when the father spied that form,
Yet he recognized his son as emerging from a storm.

Clutching his cane he hobbled down the road,
To share his son's burden of his obviously sinful load,
He fell on his neck with a welcoming kiss,
Embraced him with love and forgiving bliss.

The father refused his son's servanthood request,
But demanded a servant fetch a robe of the very best,
To put it on him together with a ring on his hand,
Plus some shoes on his feet, his joyful command.

"Bring the fatted calf and quickly have it killed,
That we may eat and rejoice and all be filled,
For this, my son who was dead and was lost,
Today is alive and found, so I'll spare no cost."

This is one of my favorite parables, and this poem has already expressed quite a lot. I was deeply moved as I put it together. The truth is it will take all eternity to try to fully comprehend God's fathomless love for His children—even those who have gone astray. The decision to retrace your steps to God, with recommitment to Him is met with a loving God with outstretched arms ready to embrace us with welcome.

The Prodigal knew he was lost. He was conscious of his condition and had the presence of mind to do something about it. He decided to turn around his lifestyle and chose to forsake the mess. He would now submit to the One who is able to take care of his future.

Thank God he did. You, too, can retrace your steps if you have gone astray, renew your covenant with Him as you repent, confess and accept Jesus as your personal Savior from sin today. He is waiting for you.

According to Travis & Ryan (2004),….Ultimately, inner peace comes from being sufficiently relaxed and balanced within yourself that you can feel your connectedness to your family, friends, community, the planet, and any transcendent reality you may experience.

The Unjust Steward
(Luke 16: 1–13)

A rich lord had a manager o'er his business
Who was accused of poor managerial skills,
So the lord inquired into his stewardship fitness,
That he should explain any variance of the bills.

He expected to be fired in utter shame,
Should he his boss not impress,
So he thought of a plan to save his name,
And the truth he will not confess.

He summoned the debtors, all they who toil,
Asking, "How much the lord do you owe?"
The first replied "one hundred measures of oil"
"Quick.... write fifty here... he will not know."

And to another he spoke so charmingly sweet,
"Do you owe the boss anything more?"
"Oh yes," he replied, "a hundred measures of wheat"
"Here... take this bill...and write only fourscore."

The rich lord came and into the books he looked,
And found a rather impressive record.
He did not know that the books were "cooked"
And that everything was not above board.

He showered praises on that unjust steward,
Complimenting him for being so wise,
For he saved his job with a generous reward
By deceitful means he did devise.

Let he who has little be faithful with his trust,
And be faithful in the very much too,
For he who in little is very unjust,
Will mismanage a windfall to rue.

The Rich Man and Lazarus
(Luke 16: 19–31)

The rich man was well-dressed,
Lots of food to eat,
Living in his mansion blessed–
But the beggar man Lazarus,
Crawling on his feet,
Full of sores and oozing pus,
Just cried for the crumbs.

Well, the beggar died one day.
Angels took him to Abram's bosom.
The rich man also passed away–
Into hell he sadly reached.
With tormenting flames and pains therefrom,
To Abraham he beseeched
For Lazarus to get him some water.

Abraham said, "Son, remember well,
In your life you never cared.
Lazarus endured an earthly hell—
He was never comforted,
His pains you never spared.
Now, you are tormented
In your final hell."

"Besides, this gulf is great
Between you and us.
So bear your wretched fate—
For here no contact can be made
As no one can cross."
Eternally lost, I'm afraid,
No more chances after death.

This parable of Lazarus teaches us several lessons that should open our eyes to the implications of life here and in the hereafter.

Firstly, we note that the poor will always be among us. Secondly, there will be the rich or better privileged, broadly speaking. Thirdly, while we are alive here on earth, this is the time and opportunity to do for others what we can do so as to help alleviate their unfortunate plight. After death it is impossible.

Jesus here was using figurative language to reach an audience in His day who believed that there was some consciousness after death. But the Bible clearly states this is not so. Supporting texts include Psalms 146:4; Ecclesiastes 9:5–7; Ecclesiastes 12; 7. Lazarus in Abraham's bosom was a *symbol* of compassion and refuge which the Jews understood very well.

That mean, rich man ended up tormented in raging flames of fire in hell. Again, the dialog between him and Abraham is *figurative,* for his tongue would have been so scorched thus eradicating the idea of him being able to talk and beg Abraham to send Lazarus for water to place on his tongue. Even then, what relief could a drop of water bring to his burning body?

Jesus, in this parable, was careful to mention that there was a great gulf fixed between them, so that no contact whatever could be made. Even if verbal contact were *actually* possible, the great span of the gulf, plus the sound of the raging fires would mean that the rich man would have to talk very loudly even though his entire body is on fire.

Some people take this parable in a literal sense to support the notion that when a "good' person dies, he or she goes straight to heaven immediately. As pointed out before, this is impossible because it will imply that those who are not "good' will go straightway to a burning hell now. Then, if heaven is way beyond the skies above, hell is close by and burning furiously right now. And a lot of desperate cries are heard across the gulf between heaven and hell!

So we are left to assume that the saved in heaven are very sad that they cannot offer help. And in heaven there is to be no sadness or crying!.... We cannot take the parable literally. The great truth from the parable is that while we are alive today, now is the time to do good, for after death, it will be too late.

Amidst the turmoil and strife…Wellness is guaranteed life…From the Source of life, Jesus…

"In Him we live and move and have our being" (Acts 17:28).
"…I am come that they might have life, and that they might have it more abundantly." (John 10:10).

The Unprofitable Servant
(Luke 17: 7–10)

Suppose your servant is out all day,
Plowing or looking after the sheep,
But at nightfall he comes in to stay,
For some rest and a good night's sleep.

But before you invite him to come and eat,
He commands, "Get me my evening meal,
Complete with drink and tasty meat,
And wait 'till I'm done with the deal."

Sometimes after completing our assigned tasks,
We engage such unworthy servanthood,
For we only do what our Master asks,
Yet craves his very best good.

Travelers on the way to God's eternal kingdom are to be considerate of and generous to their elders and superiors in the name of the Lord. Acting out of character, compounded with haughtiness and ostentatiousness, can be self-defeating in the long run. While some people claim that vociferous demands, with some intimidation maybe, is the only way to get action, the way of Godly peace is still God's way.

The Persistent Widow
(Luke 18: 1–8)

In a certain town there lived a judge,
Nothing would make him budge–
He feared neither God nor cared about men,
To be kind, he had to think again.

Every day a widow begged of him her plea,
"Please, grant me justice against my adversary."
But he kept refusing, paying her no heed,
While she kept returning, her case to plead.

Because of her persistence he finally succumbed,
To her cries and her pains, no longer benumbed.
He granted her justice while hoping for the best
Not to see her again to give him any more stress.

Will not God grant justice to your very plight?
Who cry out to Him all day and all night?
Do you have faith to persist in prayer,
To hold on to God in your doubt and fear?

The underlying virtue in this parable is that persistence in faith pays rich dividends. When it comes to God, He welcomes our persistence in reasoning with Him. He never gets tired of us as mankind is prone to do. As a loving Father, many are the opportunities He allows us to encounter so as to help us develop resilience in character, patience and endurance in faith. Sometimes we ask God for one thing and the response seems to be anything other than that thing and we deem it to be unanswered prayer because the outcome is different from what we expected. But God has His own timeframe by which to work and it is certainly different from ours. As such, we should not grow despondent and give up too easily. Be like the widow—just continue to persist in prayer. 1 John 5:5 reminds that *"And this is the confidence that we have in him, that, if we ask any thing according to his will, he heareth us."*

The Pharisee and The Publican
(Luke 18: 9–14)

A parable spoke Jesus to the listening crowd
About trusting in self with self-righteousness,
Despising others with an air so proud,
In the name of religion and holiness.

Two men went into the temple to pray,
One a Pharisee and the other, a Publican.
Each had his bit from his heart to say,
In the presence of God, and that of man.

The Pharisee lifted his voice in prayer,
"I thank you Lord I am not as other men are"
Recommending himself so highly for all to hear,
To everyone near and to those quite afar.

"No extortioner, sinner or adulterer am I,
No, not even like this publican sinner here,
I fast twice a week and I do not lie,
Pay all my tithes when my food crops bear."

But the publican afar in a repentant poise,
Guilty of his sins would not lift his poor head,
But smiting his breast and weeping silently,
"God be merciful to me, a sinner instead."

I tell you God answered that publican's call,
While the pharisee's prayer went down the drain.
Self-exaltation is a recipe for your fall,
But humility brings blessings in its train.

The attitude of worship should be crowned with selfless love–love to God and love to man. True love for our fellow human beings will allow no room in belittling others and trying to promote oneself at the expense of others' misfortunes.

God has allowed some to occupy privileged positions in this life with the hope that such would reach out to the less fortunate so as to help ease their burdens in some little way. As brothers' and sisters' keepers, the joys of sharing and encouraging will serve to enrich lives and develop worthy characters for His kingdom.

The Bible deems all our righteousness as filthy rags and that there is none good, no not one. We are all sinners in need of God's grace. The grace of God is what makes us somebody. By ourselves, we are nothing. Jesus in the life makes the difference and so we need to have that connecting relationship with Him daily. The Pharisee was lacking in this regard.

In humble repentance we should acknowledge our shortcomings and deficiencies of character and invite Him into our lives to effect that radical transformation from unworthiness to worthiness. Publicizing our accomplishments to draw attention to self rather than to God is a distraction to spiritual development.

A timely word in spiritual wellness as advanced by the apostle Paul encourages *"I beseech you therefore, brethren, by the mercies of God, that ye present your bodies a living sacrifice, holy acceptable unto God, which is your reasonable service. And be not conformed to this world: but be ye transformed by the renewing of your mind, that ye may prove what is that good, and acceptable, and perfect, will of God." (Romans 12:1, 2. KJV).*

The Pounds
(Luke 19: 11–27)

A very far country was a nobleman's destination,
A kingdom to acquire was his grand intention.
"Occupy till I come," he told his servants ten,
As he gave each a pound, hoping to see them again.

His citizens hated him for no reason at all,
Hoping from his position one day he will fall,
But he acquired the kingdom and returned to his land,
And summoned the servants before him to stand.

"How was your trading?" he inquired expectantly,
"Your pound brought me ten more!" the first said joyously,
"Well done, good servant, since in little you had such faith,
Over ten cities you shall rule, for today I make you great."

The second came saying "Thy pound gained me five!"
The master was so happy he seemed to come alive,
"Then rule over five cities" was the unexpected reward,
"What faithful endurance of a dedicated steward."

But one came saying, "Lord, here is thy pound,
I've kept it securely wrapped, laid under the ground,
For your austerity caused me fears that only seemed to grow,
Knowing that you like to reap where you will never sow."

The master was annoyed at the very poor excuse,
For slothfulness was defended with inexcusable abuse.
A deposit in a bank would've been a much better option,
For interest would've accrued to the lord's satisfaction.

Then the lord gave that pound to him with the ten,
Saying, unto him who has, to him more shall be given,
And the little that you have, if you choose not to use,
Then you'll be left with nothing, for even that you will lose.

This parable bears a striking similarity to the parable of the ten talents in Matthew, chapter 25.

The nobleman represents Jesus, our Savior, Redeemer and King, who many people still do not appreciate. But He is temporarily away, gone to prepare mansions for His faithful ones (see John 14: 1–3), and who will return soon to take them there.

In the interim, His command to us, His servants, is to be productive by using our God-given talents and resources diligently. Do not be idle and profligate, for a time of reckoning will come. We will each have to answer to God for opportunities neglected and resources wasted by shortchanging ourselves of invaluable experiences of occupational wellness. No excuse will be accepted.

We all want to hear "Well done, good and faithful servant." Mankind on this earth may fail to recognize our contributions, but better than man, is God, who is the True rewarder of our works. God sees where no man can see or understand. So, stay faithful in your duty on earth while submissive to God above. The real focus is not on the creation but on the Creator. God gives us the strength to 'occupy" till He comes and will grant us the reward in due season. Hold fast to him; His promises are sure.

My Wellness Prayer...

Lord Jesus, You are the Great Physician and I am in need of healing. Grant me the strength to submit to your counsels, and to follow your prescription for meaningful living. May your wellness principles give me hope, courage, and victory over my besetments as I accept your will today...amen.

NOTES